M000282092

KAMA
SUTRA

QUIVER

Contents

1 Nominal Kissing

2 Wrestling of the Tongues

3 Pressing Yoni Kiss

4 Kissing the Yoni Blossom

5 Sucking a Mango Fruit

6 Consuming the Lingam

7 The Kiss of the Crow

8 The Kiss of the Crow— Variation

9 The Splitting of the Bamboo

10 The Bud

11 The Outstretched Clasping Position

12 The Side-by-Side Clasping Position

13 The Conch

14 The Union Like a Crab

15 The Churning of the Cream

16 The Flag of Cupid

17 The Flower in Bloom

18 Indrani

19 The Lotus-like Position

20 The Monkey

21 The Union of Fixing a Nail

22 The Union of the Spinning Top

23 The Union Like a Swing

24 The Turning Union with Man on Top

25 The Full-Pressed Union

26 The Half-Pressed Union

27 The Packed Union

28 The Yawning Position

29 The Yawning Position—
Variation

30 The Widely-Opened
Position

31 The Wife of Indra

32 The Amazon

33 The Feet Yoke

34 The Knot of Fame

35 The Lotus

36 The Peacock

37 The Swing

38 The Trapeze

39 The Union Like a
Pair of Tongs

40 The Tortoise

41 The Peddling Tortoise

42 The Yab Yum Position

43 The Ass

44 The Cat

45 The Congress of
the Cow

46 The Rutting of
the Deer

47 The Dog

48 The Pressing of the
Elephant

49 The Congress of the
Elephant

50 Inversion

51 One Knot

52 The Rhino

Introduction

WHAT IS THE KAMA SUTRA?

The Kama Sutra is an ancient Indian text that suggested lifestyle customs and systems to create a specific type of respectful and interactive society based on virtue, wealth, and love. Loosely translated, Kama Sutra means "rules of love." The "arts" described in the Kama Sutra were taught in various phases to children and young adults so that lovers would know how to please each other.

Contrary to popular belief, the arts are not all about sexual positions. In fact, sex is only one of the arts. Other arts include daily activities, such as hygiene, farming, housekeeping, sewing, and child care, as well as fine arts, such as music, painting, poetry, and dance.

There are varying ideas about sex and the Kama Sutra, and those notions have been assumed and speculated about for centuries. The Kama Sutra itself is based on spiritual ideas rooted in Eastern religions. When it comes to the sexual ideas presented in the text, people became confused. And it's no wonder. The Kama Sutra went underground for a long time. Only now that the text has become mainstreamed are there several translations and interpretations about what, exactly, it means. Some people believe the Kama Sutra is only about sexual positions. Other people realize there are specific ideas about fore- and after-play. In any relationship, understanding and compromise can go a long way. Communication is crucial to any relationship. It's important to talk about what you want, what you desire, and how you can make things better for each other. Keeping your partner satisfied in the bedroom increases the likelihood of a smoother life outside the bedroom, too. Remember, you are sexual partners in all aspects of your lives, and you should constantly respect and show affection for one another. Your sexual life will carry through in everything that you do—from preparing a meal to washing the car. With the respect and validation you receive in a satisfying sexual relationship, you may find your life as a whole, as well as within the partnership, grow more vital and interesting.

For those wishing to understand more about the Kama Sutra, there are many books on the subject, as well as Internet sites.

WHO IS THIS BOOK FOR?

This book has been created for the average couple— a couple that has been together long enough to be fully comfortable with one another. Age, weight, color, and race are not factors here. What is important is that you treat your body well, as the Kama Sutra calls for stamina, flexibility, and even sex drive. You and your partner should be comfortable with each other—as you can see, a woman needs to trust her man completely while he holds her upside down or suspended in the air. Likewise, a man needs to trust his woman to communicate with him if she's being hurt, needs more time to warm up, or if her leg is sore.

I am a woman in her forties, of average weight and average height. I have tried all fifty-two positions selected here and could get into nearly every position as required. Admittedly, some positions, due to the weight and flexibility limitations of my partner and I, wouldn't rank as first choice for endless pleasure.

I have included positions for people of any size and weight. With some positions, yoga or ballet training will help to rev up your flexibility. It is important to remember that even our beautiful models couldn't successfully manipulate themselves completely into some of the ancient complex positions, so don't get frustrated. Do whatever works best for you and have fun!

WHY I CREATED THIS BOOK

I created this book to bring joy and fun to a couple's sex life. It is an informational tool intended to open the door to candid conversation between man and woman.

Some of the positions are animal-like, and this is to invite a sense of play between partners. These positions help remind us not to take life so seriously. Some of the positions have one partner dominant over the other. Some positions inspire laughter as the partners try to manipulate their bodies, and laughter is one of the biggest stress releases in the world. If you can combine sex and laughter, chances are good you will be able to successfully build a solid relationship with one another.

Remember, it's not important that you mimic these positions perfectly. The idea is for you to try new and different positions, techniques, and angles in an effort to please each other.

The average couple gets hooked on an idea — or if you're lucky, two — in the bedroom and this becomes routine. After all, if we've figured out how to fit oat each other's boat and we're happy, why mess with perfection?

But people get bored. Even if you've found the magic button, knee-knocking, head-spinning, body-slamming positions that work for you, how long do you think it will be before you grow tired of doing the same old thing?

HOW TO USE THE BOOK

Use these positions however you like — with toys, costumes, ropes, furniture, pillows, etc.— or wherever your imagination takes you.

You can have your partner choose one for a night's exploration or you can simply add some new material into your usual routine each week. Try the positions in the order presented or try them at random. Choose a missionary, rear-entry, or standing position in each play session. Or perfect your technique with one position before moving onto the next.

It's important to try to understand why each position is different and also to attempt to perform it as closely as described because there are nuances in some positions where you don't realize how exciting they are until you are actually doing them.

Remember, too, that thrusting isn't the key to every position. Some positions require "milking" or "squeezing" by the woman and some positions require gentle rocking, sliding, or undulating. Try different ways of feeling your bodies connect.

Throughout the book, specific terminology from the Kama Sutra is used to describe different sex organs. The penis is referred to as the lingam, the female outer genitalia or lips are referred to as the yoni, and the female outer genitalia or lips with the clitoris are referred to as the *flowering lotus*.

PREPARATION

Your bedroom is your sanctuary. Try to keep it private and comfortable for adult play. Keep the room clean and uncluttered. Use different scented oils or candles to inspire lust and love.

Your body is your main play toy. Some of the cards suggest exercises and breathing techniques that will loosen the body up and inspire greater flexibility. Stretching before—and after—a vigorous encounter can help prevent pulling muscles.

When trying new techniques or experimenting with different types of sex games, always be respectful of each other. Never force your partner to try something they are reluctant to do.

So, how many positions are there in the Kama Sutra? Opinions vary, but I've read that there are more than 500 positions. If you pay attention to the subtleties, you're guaranteed hours of excitement and a lifetime of satisfaction.

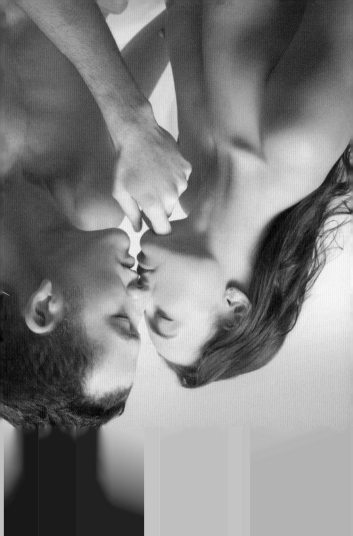

Kissing is one of the most enjoyed pleasures in the Kama Sutra. In fact, there are endless ways of kissing your lover when you start to combine methods. Some people fall into a style of kissing and use it on a regular basis, while others like to experiment with their lips and tongues. Use kissing to flirt, comfort, tease, and show intent. Try kissing with your eyes open. Use your hands to explore each other's bodies while pressing your hearts together. Breathe in unison as your lips kiss and dance with each other.

TYPES OF KISSES

Nominal	Let only the lips touch.
Throbbing	When the lips touch, "pulse" the bottom lip.
Touching	Touch your lover's lips with your tongue like a snake, then kiss.
Straight	Nominal kiss with bodies and lips "straight on," tilt only for noses.
Bent	Deep-locking kiss with tongues penetrating fully, hand cupping neck.
Turned	Place hands on lover's face to tilt up, kiss slowly with passion.
Pressed	Hold lover's lower lip, gently touch lip with tongue, then kiss fully.
Upper lip	Suck the upper lip of your lover while your lower lip is sucked.
Clasping	Take lovers lips into own, add tongue for more fun.
Wrestling	Wrestle with each other's tongues, involve gums, teeth, and lips.

KISSING ENHANCEMENT

Both partners should keep their lips soft and supple by using creams. Men should keep their faces freshly shaved and moisturized. And everyone appreciates fresh breath, so remember to carry breath mints.

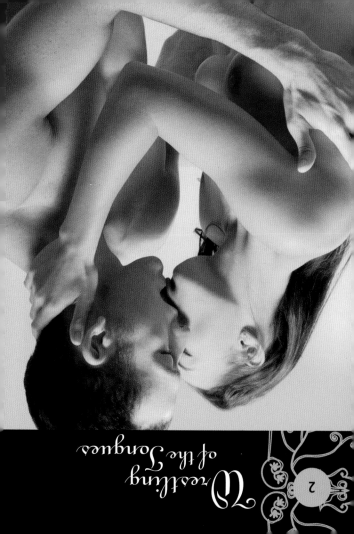

Wrestling of the Tongues

2

Kissing is always enjoyable and erotic and can be done before, during, and after sex. According to the Kama Sutra, kissing is of four kinds or styles, each of which is appropriate for a different part or parts of the body. Remember, any part of the body with flesh will benefit from your lover's kiss. Take the time to explore one another by kissing the eyelids, forehead, neck, fingers, and toes.

STYLES OF KISSING

STYLE	BODY PART	TECHNIQUE
Soft kiss	Breasts, crevices	Gentle nips, licking
Moderate kiss	Cheeks, breast, hips, belly	Nibble with teeth
Full-on kiss	Whole body	Kissing, licking curves
Contracted kiss	Lips, body	Scratch nails along body

FUNCTIONAL KISSING

Kiss That Kindles Love	The woman watches her man's face while he sleeps. She kisses him on the face, waking him for sexual adventure.
Kiss That Turns Away	If your partner is working too hard, sneak up behind and gently kiss him or her. This kiss turns your lover's attention towards you and away from work.
Kiss That Awakens	When the man returns home late, he kisses his woman to awaken her for sex. The woman can pretend to be asleep to add thrill to the chase.
Kiss That Shows Intent	Kiss your lover's reflection on the mirror. This shows desire.
Transferred Kiss	Kiss a picture of your lover, an object, or imagine someone that the lover desires while watching your lover with inviting eyes. This promotes the desire to be kissed for real.
Demonstrative Kiss	If you want to kiss someone, kiss his or her

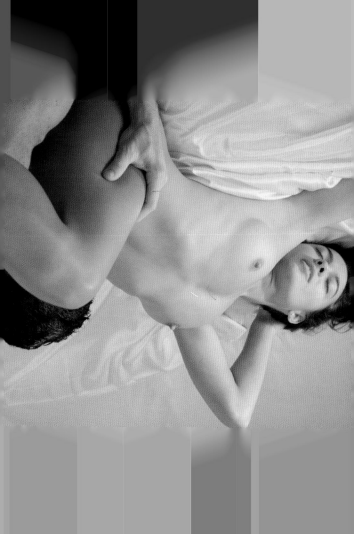

The woman lies on the edge of the bed with her legs spread, as the man kneels on the floor, his head between her legs. He presses her yoni with his lips, like a kiss. He then stimulates her belly, breasts, and thighs with his hands as he kisses her, without using his tongue, several times—this shows respect and is also great foreplay.

VOCABULARY
In the Kama Sutra, some of the sex organs are called by different names.

SEX ORGAN	KAMA SUTRA TERMINOLOGY
Penis	Lingam
Female outer genitalia or lips	Yoni
Outer genitalia or lips with the clitoris	Flowering lotus

Historical Fact

In Eastern cultures, the yoni is treated with great respect and reverence. Women are respected for their work, as well as for being the givers of life. Stimulation of the lotus releases sexual energy, which flows out in juices. Men drink these juices to fill themselves with sexual energy and power.

YONI KISSES, PART ONE

Outer yoni tongue strokes	Gently open the yoni while gently kissing, licking, and probing with the tongue.
	◄◄◄
Inner yoni tongue strokes	Open the outer labia and lick the inner lips.

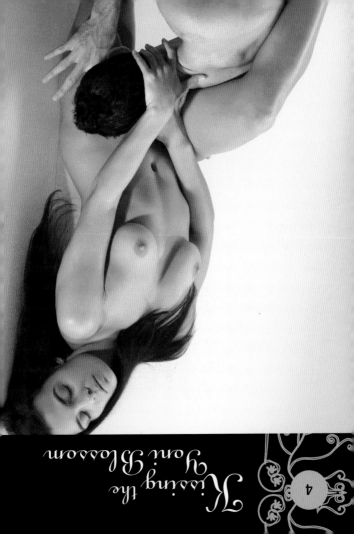

Kissing the Your Blossom

4

The woman stands with her legs apart as the man kneels on the floor between her legs, holding her yoni open, exposing the clitoris. With his tongue, he gently strokes upward along her shaft, licking either side of her clitoris in an upward fashion. Long, sensual sucks on her yoni will drive her wild. Kissing the Yoni Blossom can also be done with the woman sitting or lying down.

YONI KISSES, PART TWO

Flutter of the Butterfly	Kiss the yoni while softly fluttering the tongue along the shaft of the clitoris.
Kissing the Blossom	Lick the clitoris on either side of the shaft. Run the **Yoni** tongue across the head and give long, sensual sucks to her yoni.
Sucking the Yoni Blossom	Tenderly suck the clitoris in a gentle, tender manner; caress the clitoris with the tongue.
Kiss of the Penetrating Tongue	Begin with shallow, flicking licks of the yoni. Penetrate and withdraw the tongue, increasing pressure. As excitement increases, thrust the tongue deeper.
Drinking from the Fountain of Life	Enjoy the juices that flow from the yoni, celebrating sexual energy as well as the energy of life. If the G-spot is correctly stimulated, most women have the ability to ejaculate.

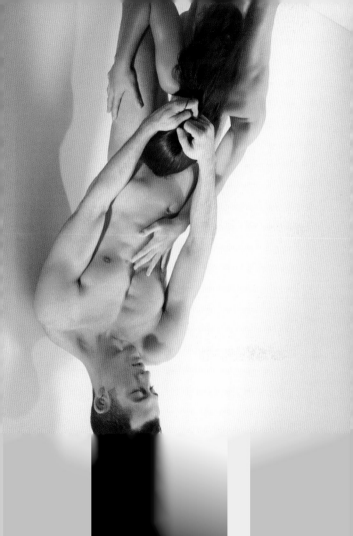

The woman takes the man's lingam halfway into her mouth, sucking with intense pressure—similar to sucking on a lollipop or ripe mango. She can alternate sensations by opening her mouth and sucking gently.

This position may be performed sitting, standing, or lying down. The woman may kneel before her man as she takes his lingam into her mouth, and the man can also lean against a wall or pillar for support. Using eye contact and stroking the woman's hair, the man can signal his level of enjoyment and pleasure. Eye contact from the woman not only enhances the level of enjoyment and pleasure, but also gives him a sense of power.

LINGAM KISSES, PART ONE

Nominal Lingam Kiss	The woman holds his lingam in her hand and places her lips around it. Moving his lingam in her mouth, she uses her lips to press and release him, pulling away her mouth.
Side Nibbling Lingam Kiss	The woman holds his lingam with her fingers as she kisses and nibbles in a gentle manner, up and down the sides. For added pleasure, she can change the pressure of her kisses.
Outside Pressing Lingam Kiss	The woman presses the head of his lingam with closed lips. She kisses it while gently sucking it like a straw.
Inside Pressing Lingam Kiss	The woman puts his lingam into her mouth, keeping her lips firm and sucking his lingam with great force, then slowly withdraws it from her mouth.
Sucking a Mango	The woman takes his lingam halfway into her mouth and sucks.

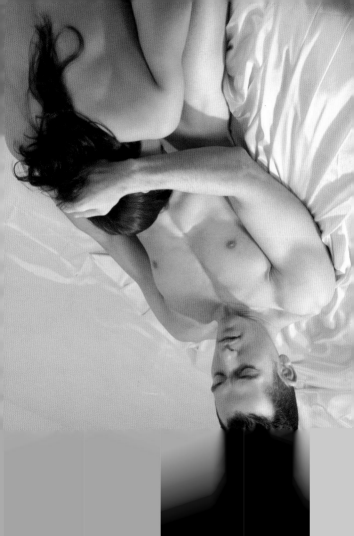

In this position, the woman takes the man's lingam fully into her mouth (also known as "deep-throat").

Men who are well endowed can prove to be a challenge for some women. Try experimenting with different positions—fellatio can be performed while kneeling before your lover as he sits on the edge of the bed, he can lean against a wall, or you can both lie down. To see which way works best for sliding the man's lingam as far down the throat as you're comfortable with, try having him stand at the end of the bed as you lie on either your stomach or your back. If you sit in a rocking chair while he stands before you, the gentle rocking may entice his lingam to slip further down your throat.

TRAINING EXERCISE

Practice opening the back of the throat by pretending to yawn. Remember to breathe deeply and slowly through your nose. Practice holding your breath and relaxing your throat at the same time so that you can feel relaxed when performing fellatio.

LINGAM KISSES, PART TWO

Kiss the Lingam	Holding the lingam firmly in her hand, the woman kisses the head as she would his lower lip, pressing and moving her lips in a gentle manner.
Lingam Tongue Stroke	The woman holds the man's lingam in her hand, licking and stroking him with her tongue. She can flick and press his frenulum—the triangular area of skin on the underside of the lingam—or anywhere else he enjoys.
Consuming the Lingam	The lingam is fully consumed by the mouth and throat.

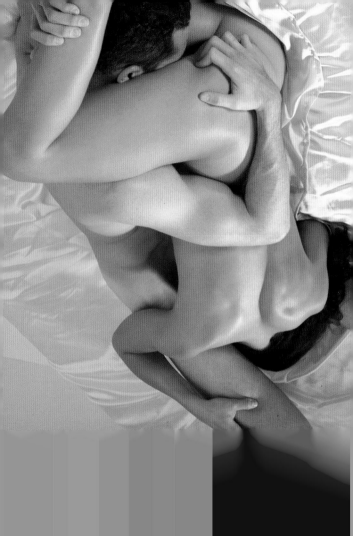

The Kiss of the Crow is, in fact, what most people know as the "69" position, in which lovers give and receive oral sex at the same time. With both lovers lying down on the bed, or on their sides, their faces are between each other's legs. It can take some maneuvering for a couple to determine which position provides the best comfort and access, but once in place, the couple can stimulate each other's genitals with lips, tongues, and fingers.

For people who are shy about giving or receiving oral sex, the Kiss of the Crow is a great way to experiment as there is no pressure to perform solo—both of you are pleasing each other at the same time. An added benefit to the Kiss of the Crow is that partners can mirror each other's actions and excitement level.

Don't worry about achieving perfect coordination. It's absolutely fine if your partner is licking you fast while you're licking slowly, or if one of you stops to enjoy the sensations for a moment.

It is a good thing if the woman can climax during oral sex, since many women may have difficulty reaching orgasm during intercourse. Many times, orgasms from oral sex are stronger then orgasms from intercourse, no matter what gender you are. Additionally, oral sex is safer than intercourse as it cannot lead to pregnancy.

SEDUCTIONS

You can try different sensations by sucking on ice cubes or a mint before oral sex. However, you should be aware that some types of toothpastes and mouthwashes may be more irritating to sensitive genital tissues than enjoyable.

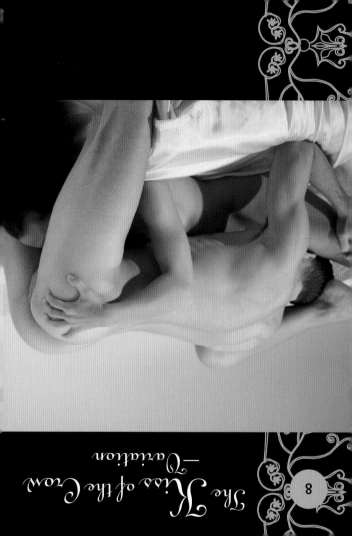

The Kiss of the Crow
—Temptation

The woman lies on the bed with her head hanging over the side, keeping her legs either bent or straight, but spread open. The man stands at her head, placing his lingam into her mouth, and then bends over to kiss her yoni.

There are many ways to play with this position. For instance, the man can tuck his hands under the woman's buttocks and lift her so that he can lick her from yoni to buttocks or he can kiss her thighs—teasing and playing with her the entire time.

Some women enjoy the use of fingers or a toy while receiving oral sex. The man can use these to stimulate her G-spot while sucking on her clitoris.

The woman can grip her man's buttocks and thighs while she's sucking and licking his lingam and testicles. She can even give love taps and slaps on his butt, or cup her hands around his testicles.

The man can reach between his legs, and cradle the woman's head in his hands to guide her pacing—making it faster or slower. Cradling her head also helps the woman to bob her head and reduces possible neck strain. To ease things for the man, the woman may want to hold her own yoni open while the man is stimulating her.

No matter which way you maneuver it, this position is a lot of fun and takes the body weight off of both parties.

SEDUCTION

With the man standing at the end of the bed and the woman lying on her back with her head off the bed, deep-throating might be much easier.

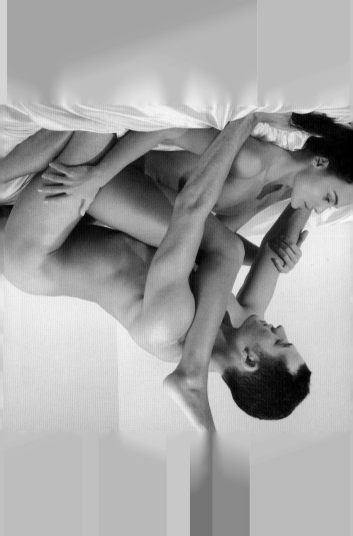

The woman lies on her back with her legs bent as the man kneels over her, placing one hand on each side of her head. The woman raises one leg and places it over his shoulder. She straightens her other leg along the bed. The man straightens the same leg as the woman on the same side (i.e., his left, her right). His tucked leg is the same one that the woman has over his shoulder (i.e., his right, her left).

TYPES OF YONIS

Doe   Petite with a gentle manner, her yoni is tight and shallow.

Mare   Stout with a wild personality and a flair for the unusual, her yoni is full and sensuous.

Elephant   Tall and big-boned with a ruddy or radiant complexion, her yoni is wide and deep.

TYPES OF LINGAMS

Hare   A small and lively body with a gentle voice and manner, his lingam is about three inches long when erect.

Bull   Sturdy in build and with a good temperament, his lingam is thick and about four inches long when erect.

Stallion   Tall, muscular, adventurous, and fun, his lingam is about six inches when erect.

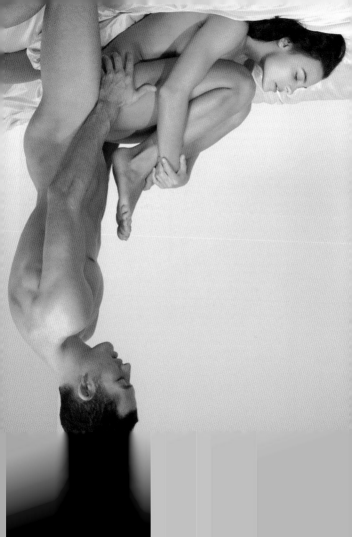

The woman lies on her back, tucking her knees up to her breasts so the yoni is exposed. She holds her knees with her arms or hands as the man sits up straight on his knees to penetrate her.

In this position, the woman can feel vulnerable with her yoni exposed. The man may wish to rub and suck on her yoni blossom to stimulate her. The man should look into her eyes as he penetrates her.

A word of caution: a stallion penetrating a doe (see #9) should take care as this position can be very deep for some women.

The Kama Sutra offers several different types of thrusting. Everyone gets hooked on their favorite rhythms and routines. Sometimes it's easy to forget there are other ways to move. Alternate your technique and remember that there is more than one way to thrust.

THE WORK OF THE MAN, PART ONE

Churning
The man holds his lingam in his hand and swirls it around inside her yoni, as if he were churning butter. Be careful not to churn too wide.

>-+-

Rubbing
The woman can lie on her back with a pillow under her buttocks, or she can sit on the edge of the bed while the man stands or kneels at the edge, penetrating her so his lingam rubs against the bottom of her vagina and perineum. This type of thrusting provides a pleasurable downward pressure.

>-+-

Moving Forward
The man puts his lingam in the woman's yoni and moves straight forward—in and out. The thrust can be varied in both pace and power.

>-+-

Piercing
The woman lies on her back as the man enters her so his lingam strokes her clitoris with each thrust.

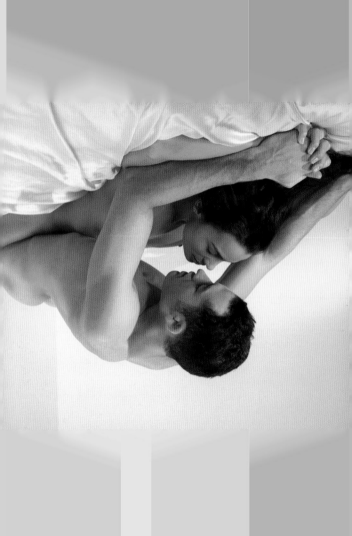

The woman lies flat on her back with her arms straight above her head and her legs straight out and apart. The man lies fully extended on top of her, covering her body, with his thighs inside of hers. He places his lingam in her yoni as they hold hands and kiss passionately.

THE WORK OF THE MAN, PART TWO

Pressing	The man inserts his lingam as far into the woman's yoni as he can and holds it there. The longer he stays there, the more pleasure the couple will experience.

——✦——

The Blow the Boar	The man angles his body so he is thrusting against only of one side of the woman's yoni, then changes angles and thrusts to the other side.

——✦——

The Blow of the Bull	The man enters and fills the yoni from all angles.

——✦——

The Sporting of the Sparrow	The man moves his lingam up and down inside the woman's yoni, increasing in pace until reaching mutual pleasure.

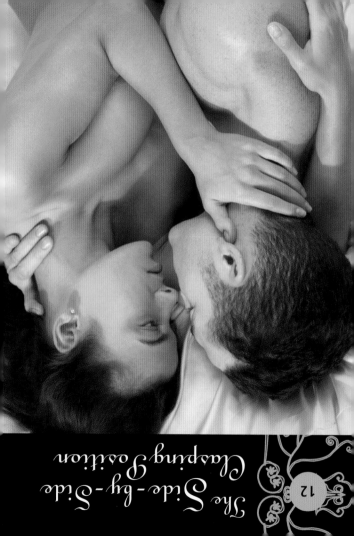

The Side-by-Side
Clasping Position

The woman lies on her right side with the man lying on his left side. They wrap their arms around each other as they kiss and stare into each other's eyes, enjoying the full body contact as the man puts his lingam into her yoni.

Historical Fact

In ancient India, the woman always stood or sat to the right of her man in daily life. This was done in adherence to the belief that feminine energy, called Shakti, is on the right side of masculine energy, called Shiva, at all times—except during sexual activity. The exchange of sides represents the shifting energies, or gears, from everyday life to the heightened awareness of sensual delight.

It's important to recognize the difference between masculine and feminine energies—particularly the difference between the amount of time it takes for man and woman to each feel satisfied. Timing is a challenge for sexual adventures partly because it takes less time for a man to become aroused, while women take longer to become aroused and are often still aroused following climax. Being aware of our differences can help us learn how to better please

NINE TYPES OF TIMING

High Compatibility		Low Compatibility		Very Low Compatibility	
◄◄―		◄◄―		◄◄―	
MAN	WOMAN	MAN	WOMAN	MAN	WOMAN
short ------- short		short -------- moderate		short ------- long	
moderate --- moderate		moderate --- short		long --------- short	
long --------- long		moderate --- long		long --------- moderate	

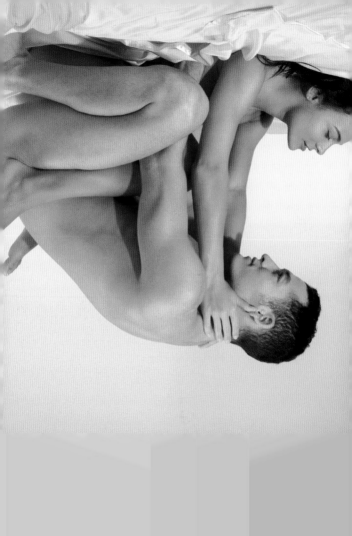

The woman lies on her back and draws her knees up to her chest. The man squats over her and puts his lingam into her yoni, clamps his thighs around hers, and rides her.

For better support and movement, the man can hold his partner by the hips or buttocks. The woman can also hold her legs up with her hands. Hares paired with elephants (see #9) may wish to use pillows to raise the woman's pelvis and buttocks higher.

This position can be quite pleasurable as it provides deeper penetration and allows for the G-spot to easily be found and stimulated. The woman may also wish to stimulate her clitoris with her fingers or a little vibrator, if she isn't already holding up her legs with her hands.

SEDUCTIONS

Pillows, cushions, and even bunched-up sheets can enhance a session by providing more choices of angles. (There are also products designed specifically for exploring different intercourse positions.) Using pillows underneath the woman's pelvis, hips, thighs, or lower back can help angle her, allowing her to relax and let the pillows do the work. And don't forget pillow support for necks, shoulders, and arms.

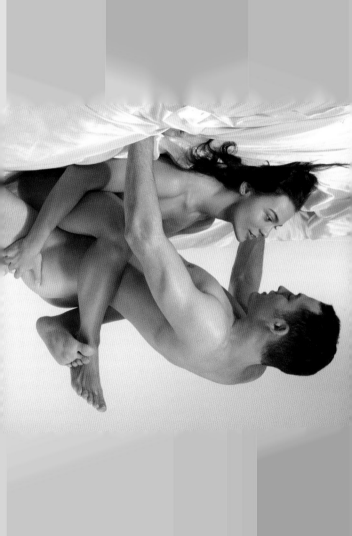

The woman lies on her back, crossing her legs and drawing them up toward her stomach. The man kneels before her with his knees set widely apart. He can keep his legs tucked under him or he can bend them behind him. If the woman chooses, she can wrap her legs around the man's waist, keeping them curled as much as possible. The man keeps his back straight as he bends slightly over her, holding her by her knees or putting his hands on the bed as he enters her.

MASSAGE

Humans love to be touched and stroked. Try giving each other loving massages before a sexual encounter—or anytime for that matter. Massage can release tension, build intimacy, and activate acupuncture points that release pleasure and pain.

Massage is best done in dim lighting or candlelight to help create a relaxing and sensual atmosphere. Before a massage, the masseur or masseuse should rub his or her hands together lightly and rapidly, activating the hand chakra points. When the hands are tingling and warm, it is time to begin.

Massage feels best when using lotion or oil. There are many types of oils and lotions sold at specialty shops, health food stores, and sex stores. As an added, thoughtful touch, try warming the oil in a bowl of warm water before starting.

If you are massaging a man, you can use oil-based or water-based products. However, keep in mind that if you are massaging a woman, use only water-based products, as oil-based products could lead to a vaginal infection.

The Churning of the Cream

The woman lies on her back and pulls her legs as far over her head as she can. The man squats above her, holding her thighs back as he penetrates her. Remember to breathe deeply while getting into and holding this position.

The woman can spread her arms on either side for balance.

Rather than resting his weight on the woman, the man uses his own thigh muscles and feet for balance. His hands hold her thighs open both for his own balance, and for deep penetration.

Since this position allows for deep penetration, this works well for a hare paired with an elephant (see #9). If a man is a stallion, he needs to be careful and thoughtful—especially if his partner is a doe. Women with large stomachs and/or large breasts may find this position difficult.

TRAINING EXERCISES FOR HER

Deep breathing is the key to performing a position such as this. In fact, you can practice this move by yourself—especially as it's a good yoga move that stretches the back. Lying on your back, bring your legs as far back over your head as you can. You can use your hands to help push yourself back or you can keep them out to the side for balance, breathing deeply as you hold the position. With every exhale, try to stretch your legs back a little more.

Over time, your flexibility will increase and you'll be amazed how far you can stretch—eventually, you may even be able to put your knees by your ears or keep your legs out straight.

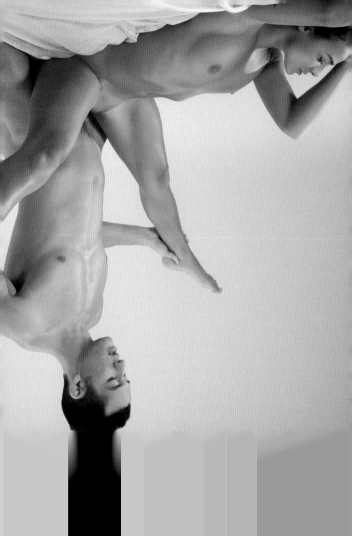

The woman lies on her back as the man kneels in front of her. The man takes one of her ankles in each of his hands. He lifts her legs so that her thighs are spread open as he penetrates her.

This position seems simple, yet it can provide great pleasure in areas that aren't normally reached in other, more traditional positions. This position can also be enhanced if the woman includes some self-pleasure—she can use her fingers or a vibrator to provide extra clitoral stimulation.

SEDUCTIONS

Men are visual creatures—this is, in part, why men's magazines and Internet pornography are so successful—pictures and visuals are immediate. Romance your man by sending him naked pictures of yourself or have a racy portrait painted of yourself for his birthday.

To provide visual stimulation for your man, play with your breasts. If you have large breasts, try sucking on your own nipples. Kneading your breasts or fiddling with your nipples by pinching and stretching them will certainly capture your lover's attention.

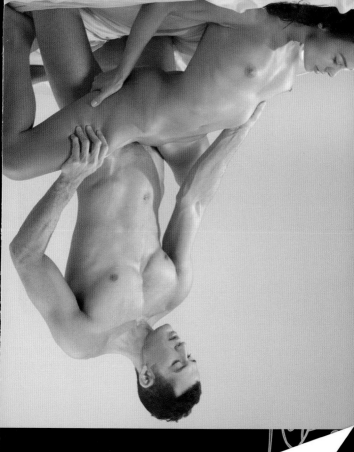

The Flower in Bloom

The woman lies on her back, placing her palms beneath her bottom and arching her yoni toward the ceiling. Spreading her thighs as wide apart as she can, she keeps her feet as close to her hips as possible. The man can sit in front of her with his legs straight out or he can kneel or crouch between her legs as he enters her.

Caressing the woman's breasts and gripping and pinching her thighs and legs can add extra pleasure. Always use eye contact to gauge each other's excitement.

THE WORK OF THE WOMAN

In many positions, the work of the woman isn't as obvious as the work of the man—nor is it as clearly defined.

THE WOMAN'S WORK

Contracting	The woman contracts her yoni, squeezing or "milking" the lingam.
Dilating	The woman dilates or "opens up" her yoni.
Normal	The woman acts normally.
Open thighs	The woman opens her thighs, especially for larger lingams.
Closed thighs	The women tightens her thighs or keeps them closer together, especially for smaller lingams.
Woman on top	The woman acts as the man, especially if the man is tired.

TRAINING EXERCISES

Kegel exercises are great for women of all types. This exercise tightens and strengthens the pelvic muscles. To feel where these muscles are, try stopping and starting the flow of urine while on the toilet.

Start by squeezing and holding for a few seconds, gradually working your way up to holding for ten seconds or more.

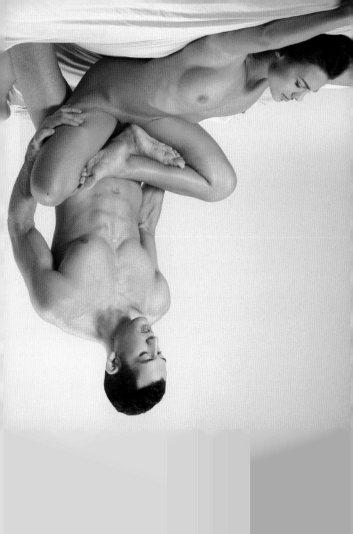

The woman lies on her back, her feet on her thighs in the lotus, or cross-legged, position. The woman can also draw her legs up as far as she can so her calves touch her thighs and her knees touch her chest. The man kneels so he can penetrate her while pressing against her thighs, opening her legs more while he thrusts. This position opens the yoni wide and tilts the pelvis up as the woman's buttocks rest against the man's thighs.

Indrani is a good position for large lingams, but keep in mind that the woman should be fully aroused before attempting this position.

MASSAGE

Massage can be part of foreplay, or it can be an experience all on its own, as it helps lovers connect with each other spiritually, mentally, and physically. Learning how to massage and incorporating it into your life will provide greater intimacy and appreciation of one another.

MASSAGE TECHNIQUES

Stroking	Muscles are grabbed and lifted in a gentle manner, then stroked.
Friction	Using thumbs and fingertips, deep circles are made in the thickest part of the muscles.
Tapotement	Fingers are pressed firmly on a muscle and the muscle is then shaken. Rhythmic tapping, stroking, chopping, and other striking movements are used.
Rocking	Massage with a gentle rocking movement. Such movement is soothing and erotic and has the ability to ease away tension and stress.

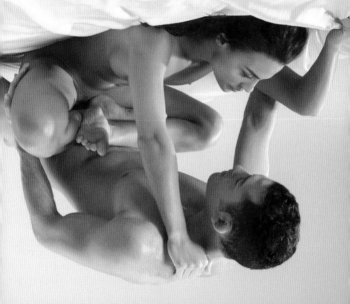

The Lotus-like Position

The woman lies on her back with her feet on her thighs in the lotus, or cross-legged, position. The man crouches over her on all fours, gently putting his lingam into her yoni.

Staring into each other's eyes in this position will give even greater intimacy. The woman can use her hands to stroke her man's face and shoulders and play with his nipples.

SEDUCTIONS

Life is busy for everyone, even more so when you have multiple jobs and children. Don't let your busy schedule put a damper on your love life. While many people believe that sex should be spontaneous, not planned, the reality is that sometimes this just isn't possible. Scheduling sex not only creates more opportunities to be intimate, but also gives you something to look forward to at the end of a hectic day.

Couples should plan a date night at least once a week. Setting aside an amount of uninterrupted time to spend together allows for you and your partner to reconnect mentally, emotionally, and physically.

On date nights—or sex nights—start foreplay early. Give kisses to one another before heading off to work, send naughty emails or make breathy phone calls to each other throughout the day, slip a note in his briefcase, or leave a note on her mirror. Touch each other when you pass in a hallway, give a little squeeze, kiss, or flirtatious glance—this will set the wheels in motion for more fun later on.

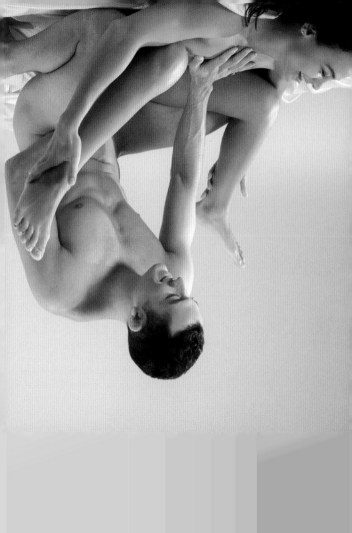

With a mischievous grin, the woman rocks onto her back, clasping her ankles in each of her hands as she raises her feet. The man crouches like a monkey between her legs. He slaps and kisses her breasts playfully as he penetrates her. If the woman is stimulated enough, happy monkeys can play in the "fountain of life energy" (see the Historical Fact in #3).

The Kama Sutra invites a sense of play. Sex is a great stress release, as is laughter. There are many animal positions in the Kama Sutra and these remind us to let ourselves relax and let go with our animal instincts. Playful positions, such as the light slapping antics of the monkey, remind us to have fun and not take life—or sex—too seriously. When exploring animal positions, inhibitions are to be checked at the door.

SEDUCTIONS

Monkeys are curious creatures and fun to mimic in the bedroom. Explore each other's bodies by tickling or play-wrestling with each other. Surely monkeys would wonder what a vibrator or dildo might do, so have some fun exploring with these in places such as the armpits, thighs, scrotum, lingam, breasts, and yoni. Throwing pillows and playing with rope can be fun, too.

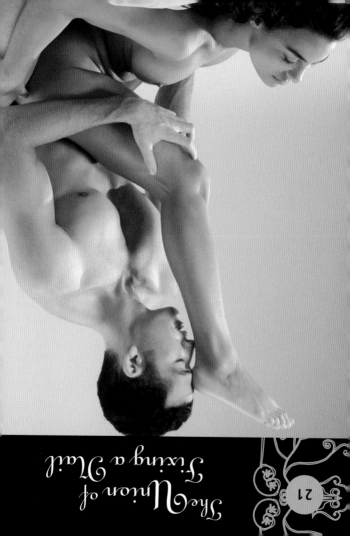

The Union of Fixing a Nail

The woman lies on her back with one leg outstretched along the bed as she raises the other leg, putting her foot on her partner's forehead, or third eye. The man kneels between her thighs, pressing against her raised leg as he thrusts.

This is a great position for eye contact. The third eye is a mystical symbol and touching it while making love can intensify the passion. The man can hold the woman's thigh, stroke her breasts, or manipulate her clitoris for added sensation.

To change sensations, the man can raise or lower the angle of his penetration and the woman can change her sensations by pressing her foot lighter or harder against her partner's forehead. The woman can stroke her lover's thighs. She can lightly scratch his skin or clasp him tightly.

PASSION

Not everyone is born with the same lust for sex. Feeble passion describes those with a low sex drive, while intense passion describes people with a high sex drive. Middling passion represents people somewhere in between. Understanding passion and timing can help a couple journey toward more interactive—and enjoyable—lovemaking.

THE NINE FORCES OF PASSION

High Compatibility		Low Compatibility		Very Low Compatibility	
⤛⤙		⤛⤙		⤛⤙	
MAN	WOMAN	MAN	WOMAN	MAN	WOMAN
Feeble ------ Feeble		Feeble ------ Middling		Feeble ------ Intense	
Middling --- Middling		Middling --- Feeble		Intense ---- Feeble	
Intense ----- Intense		Middling --- Intense		Intense ----- Middling	

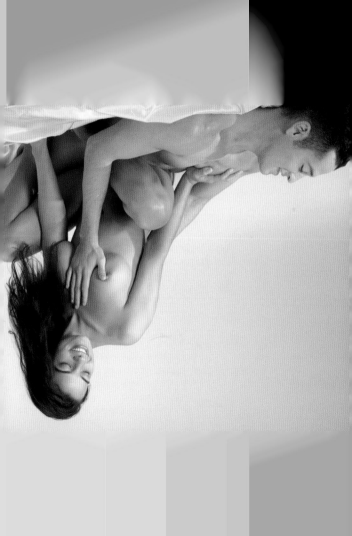

The man lies flat on the bed, his legs slightly spread. The woman squats over him, straddling his torso. Her feet are flat at his sides, with her knees up, his lingam in her yoni. She rides him, staring into his eyes while squeezing his lingam with her muscles.

Carefully, the woman turns herself to one side. To keep him inside of her, she can walk her hands over each other, and feet and legs over each other. Depending on her coordination, the man may wish to help her. Her weight and coordination will have some effect on the smoothness of the transition. Likewise, it may be more difficult for her to maneuver if the man is a stallion (see #9). Once she is sideways, she may rock, squeeze, or ride his lingam. She can also lean backward or forward.

Additionally, the woman may move herself around so that she is facing away from the man. She may put her hands on his legs for balance, or she may wish to lean backward. She may then turn to the next side and squat, rock, and ride him. Carefully, she returns to the beginning position.

This position requires some physical dexterity, cooperation, and a sense of humor. Again, this is to be a fun and comfortable position, so the woman should feel free to position herself however she likes.

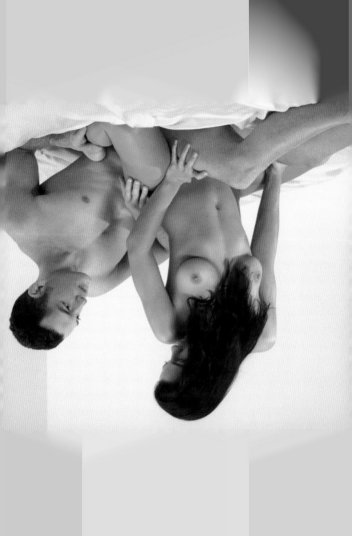

The man lies on his back, rests on his arms, or uses pillows behind his arms and back for support. The woman straddles him, facing away from him, putting her hands on his thighs or calves. Gently she rocks, or "swings" on his lingam. If the man is strong enough, he can push up his abdomen so that he is thrusting into the woman.

This position provides a much different sensation than forward-facing positions.

The woman should try to stimulate his lingam by contracting her muscles, squeezing and holding his lingam in a rhythmic manner, in sync with her swinging.

SEDUCTIONS

Atmosphere is a very important part of lovemaking. Make your bedroom your den of love and passion, and try to keep it neat and clean. Keep lighting dim, light candles, burn incense, and play music you both enjoy to create a sensual and relaxing environment.

Use high-quality sheets on your bed and always have lots of pillows handy. Remember to keep a stash of hand towels in your nightstand so you can wipe yourselves off if you get sweaty or put them down to protect the sheets.

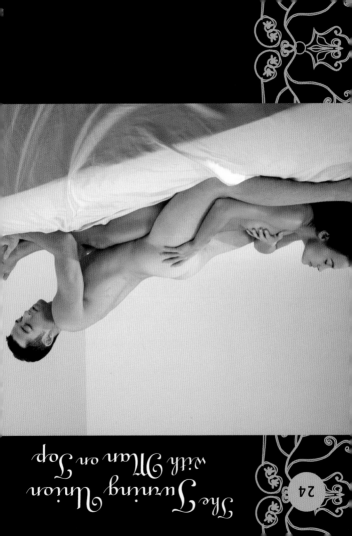

The Turning Union with Man on Top

24

The woman lies on her back with her legs out and slightly spread. The man lies on top of her and puts his lingam into her yoni (missionary style). Slowly, and carefully, he turns himself around so his head is between her feet and his feet are on either side of her shoulders. The lingam should stay in the yoni during this transition. After enjoying his woman for a while, he turns slowly around, back to the beginning.

SEDUCTIONS

The idea of this position is to go very slowly, ensuring the lingam doesn't fall out of the yoni. If the lingam does fall out, simply return to the previous position and try again.

The man will likely be unable to thrust in the turned phase of the position. The woman can squeeze her yoni or gently move underneath him. His lingam will be hitting the back of her yoni, however, and depending on size, it may be difficult for her to move at all. Rocking gently, pulsing, milking, and squeezing by the woman can all add erotic sensation for the man.

Keep in mind that when the man is turned around, this position can be uncomfortable or even painful for the woman. Feel free to stop at any time. It is always important to be aware of each other's bodies and the sensations you are feeling, never going further than you're comfortable with.

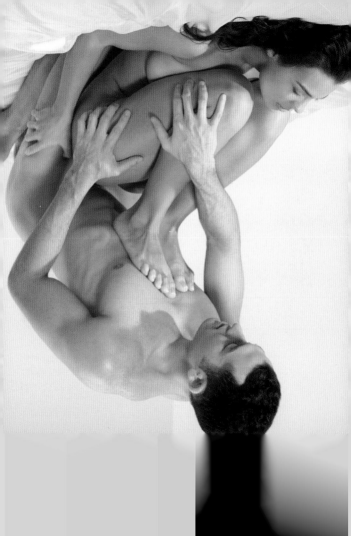

The woman lies on her back as the man kneels in front of her. Pulling her hips onto his thighs, she bends her knees and pulls her thighs to her chest. She then puts the soles of her feet against man's chest as he places his lingam into her yoni. The man stays sitting up.

The woman can change the intensity of the sensation by how hard she presses her feet against the man's chest. The use of pillows under the woman can change the angle and intensity of the position.

EMBRACES

The Kama Sutra has many types of embraces. Embraces are about touching and showing intent, and can heighten sexual excitement.

TYPES OF EMBRACES

Touching embrace	The man stands beside or in front of the woman, touching her body with his.
Rubbing embrace	Two lovers walk together as their bodies rub up against one another.
Pressing embrace	The man presses the woman up against a wall. This type of embrace can be a big turn-on for many women, as it shows the man is in charge—for the moment.
Piercing embrace	A woman may pretend to drop something in front of the man. The sight of the woman's breasts "pierces" the man and he takes hold of them.

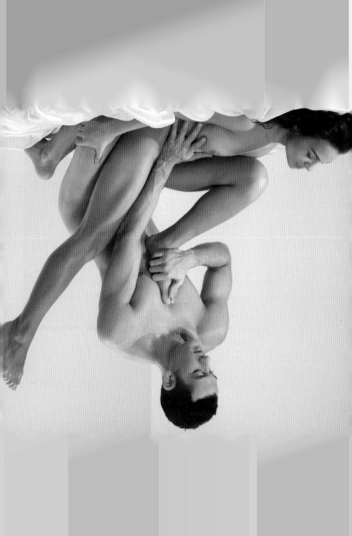

The woman lies on her back as the man kneels in front of her. He raises her hips onto his thighs and she pulls her thighs to her chest until he enters her. She places one foot on his chest and stretches the other leg straight out, over the man's thigh, moving that leg up and down.

When the woman moves her leg, she can manipulate the depth of his lingam inside of her, as well as stimulate her clitoris.

SENSUAL EMBRACES

Climbing a Tree	The man and woman stand close together with their arms around each other. The woman places one foot on the man's foot, and the other foot on his thigh—or she can loop it around his thigh as if she's climbing a tree. This is a great embrace for kissing.
Twinning of a Creeper	The man and woman stand close together, face-to-face, with arms and legs entwined. The man bends his head down to kiss the woman as they look lovingly at each other.
The Milk and Water Embrace	The man sits on the edge of a bed, on a chair, or on cushions. The woman sits on his lap with her legs wrapped around him. They embrace each other tightly, pressing their bodies into each other.
The Mixture of Sesamum Seed and Rice	The man and woman lie very close together. The man puts his leg between the woman's thighs. They embrace, wrapping their limbs tightly around each other.

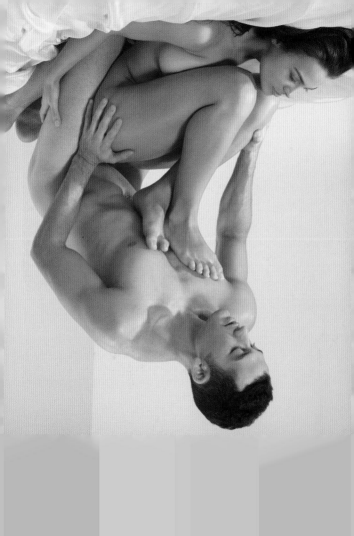

The woman lies on her back, crossing her legs at the ankles. She pulls her legs up and keeps her thighs together, close to her chest. The woman's crossed feet rest on the man's chest as he kneels before her, placing his lingam into her yoni. He can hold her buttocks or hips to create friction.

SEDUCTIONS

The woman can pinch and stroke her man's thighs or run her fingernails along his flesh. She can pull on his thighs to control his thrusts. She can also use the pressure of her feet against his chest to change the intensity of his lingam in her yoni. To leverage herself to meet his thrusts, she can put her arms on the bed.

The man can stroke her face or tug on her hair. He should look at her with loving passion, as she will feel very vulnerable.

PASSIONATE EMBRACES

Embrace of the Thighs	The man and woman can be standing, sitting, or lying down. One partner grips the other partner's thighs with his or her own.
Embrace of the Jaghana	The man presses the area between his hips and thighs against the woman, while kissing her passionately.
Embrace of the Foreheads	The man and woman touch foreheads while gazing into each other's eyes. One can kiss the other on the lips, eyes, and forehead.
Embrace of the Breasts	The man and woman can be sitting, standing, or lying down as the man presses his chest to the woman's breasts.

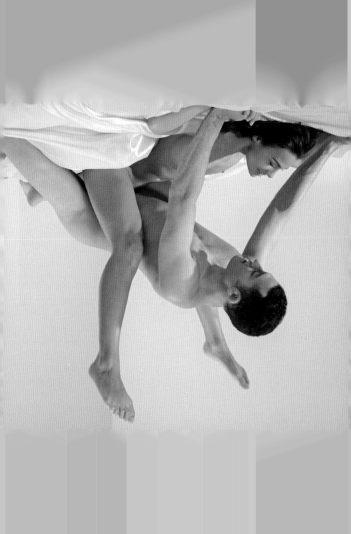

The woman lies on her back and puts her legs straight into the air. The man lies over her or kneels between her legs, placing his lingam in her yoni. The lovers press the palms of their hands together while staring into each other's eyes.

SEDUCTIONS

The woman may playfully have her lover kiss her foot or suck her toes. If this isn't appealing, she can put both of her feet on the man's shoulders.

Before intercourse begins, be certain that the woman is suitably aroused. Playing with her genitals is a surefire way to have her begging for more.

WARMING HER UP, PART ONE

Clitoral play
The man gently manipulates the hood of the woman's clitoris: gently pushing and pulling, twisting it between his fingers, or tapping it. Slowly, he works to unveil the clitoris. He teases the clitoris by flicking, tapping, and holding it between two fingers, gradually adding more constant pressure by rubbing it. He may also try going in circles or from one side to the other.

Labial play
Using a water-based lubrication, the man places his palm against his lover's vagina, fingers angled downward. Slowly he brings his hand up, hooking it into her labia. With his other hand, he plays with her inner and outer lips, tugging and stroking them.

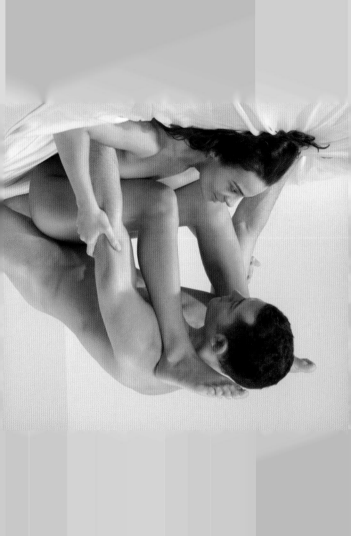

The woman lies on her back—holding her legs in the air, with her feet on each side of the man's head—as the man lies over her, almost against her thighs. For added sensation, he can squeeze her buttocks with one hand, or the couple can hold hands.

TRAINING EXERCISE

This position requires a lot of flexibility to keep the legs bent and close to the chest. A great way to build such flexibility is by doing leg stretches.

Sit on the floor and practice putting your head to your knee. Do this with your legs straight out in front of you. Try it at first with bent knees, and each day put your legs down a little more until you can touch your toes (with your fingers) without bending your knees.

Another helpful flexibility exercise is to push your legs out to either side while sitting on the floor. At first, you're not likely to get very far, but by practicing daily, you'll increase your elasticity.

The benefit of being able to keep your legs either straight or bent in the air during sex is that it will change the position of the lingam in the yoni for better penetration.

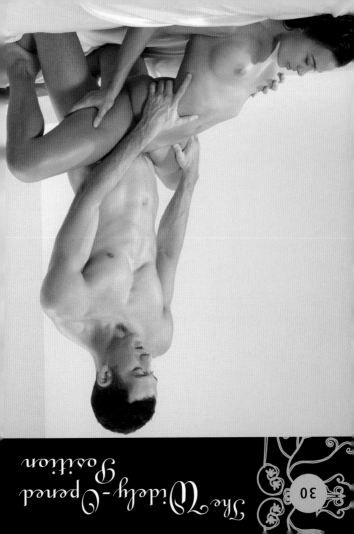

The woman lies on her back with her feet flat on the bed, then pushes her hips into the air with her knees bent and her shoulders and on the bed. The man kneels between her legs. She meets his thrusts while looking into his eyes.

SEDUCTIONS

Women who are overweight or have back problems should not attempt this position.

Using pillows under the small of the woman's back and/or her bottom takes the pressure off and helps avoid straining the back. The woman can use her hands and arms to support herself by holding her buttocks or she can have her arms flat on the bed for support. On a narrower bed, she can grip the sides for leverage.

The man can pull her hips to meet his thrusts and use his fingers to stimulate her clitoris.

TRAINING EXERCISE

This position is easily trained for by doing "Butt Ups," as we used to call them in dance class.

To do Butt Ups, lie on the floor and bend your knees. Position your feet as close to your bottom as you can and push your pelvis toward the ceiling.

Try doing a few Butt Ups, and then hold the pelvis in the air. This exercise builds up the buttocks and increases stamina. This will not only help you look great but will also help with some of the more difficult positions in the Kama Sutra.

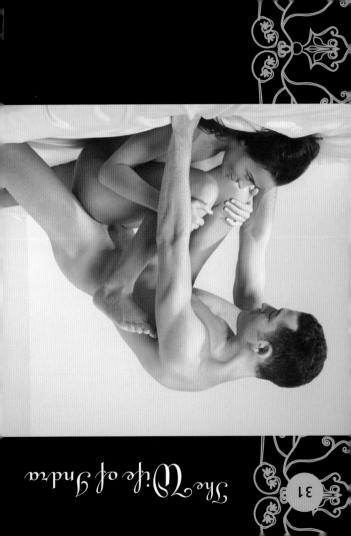

The woman lies on her back with her knees to her chest in a tuck position. She holds her knees with her hands, keeping them as close to her chest as she can. The man kneels between her legs and leans over the top of her. She puts her feet at his sides or on his navel as her buttocks rest on his pelvis. For more stimulation, the woman can flex her vaginal muscles.

This is a good position for a hare or a man with a smaller lingam (see #9). Stallions, however, should be careful, especially if the woman is a rabbit.

To do this position correctly, the woman must have strong abdominal muscles. Go easy at first. To build up to this position, try to incorporate sit-ups into your daily exercise routine.

SEDUCTION

The woman can tuck her feet into her man's armpits, gaining a bit of traction if she grips her man with her toes.

Historical Fact

Indra was a great king in Vedic history, and his wife was always trying to find new and interesting ways to have sex. She created this position for him and it was rumored to be his favorite.

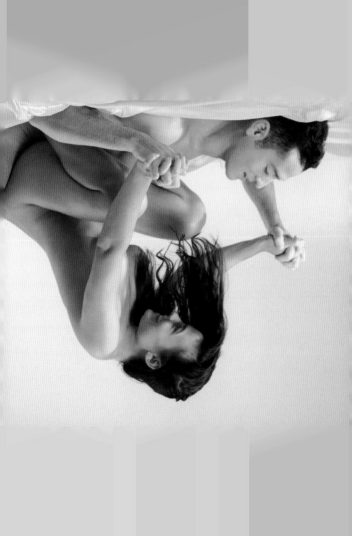

The man lies on his back with his legs bent in the air. The woman squats over him, taking his lingam into her yoni, keeping her feet squarely at his hips. He wraps his feet around her backside by hooking his ankles. They hold hands and stare into each other's eyes as she controls the movement with her thighs and body.

Play with his nipples by tweaking and teasing them or scratch his chest lightly with your fingers.

Of course, the average woman doesn't have the strength of an amazon so feel free to explore your wild side as you find other ways to balance. Try holding yourself up by leaning into the man's feet or putting your hands on his chest.

The Amazon is a good position to practice Kegels. Try to hold his lingam by clamping your vagina, while looking him in the eye. You can also slowly sway your hips to feel him swirling inside.

SEDUCTIONS

This type of position calls out for role-playing. Try dressing up in costumes.

For instance, perhaps the woman plays a superhero and the man a helpless victim. Or, the man plays a shipwrecked sailor who has stumbled upon a tribe of horny Amazonian women. Or maybe Jane has turned the tables on Tarzan. For the best results, try to find a woman-dominant scenario and be creative.

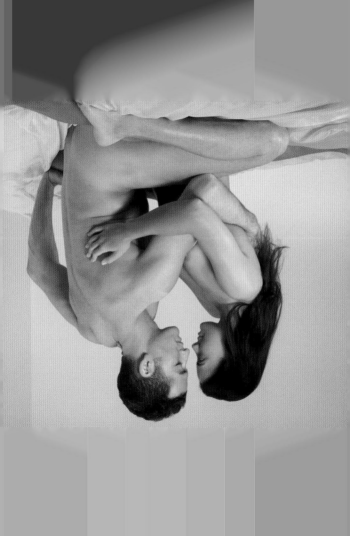

The woman sits up straight on the bed, folding one leg under her so she is sitting on it, and extending her other leg along the bed. The man sits in a similar position and places his folded leg over her extended leg and his extended leg under her folded leg as he penetrates her.

SEDUCTIONS

This position can be tricky, and requires patience and flexibility.

The lovers can wrap their arms around each other for balance, or they can each put a hand on the bed. To enhance intimacy and intensity, the couple should stare into each other's eyes.

GETTING READY

Whether a couple is getting ready for a night of passion or just a few hours of stolen time, boundaries should be set.

There should be no mention of "hot topics" such as money, jobs, or children while preparing for lovemaking. Conversation should be light and fun as the mood turns towards love. Compliments and lots of eye contact can quickly soften the atmosphere.

WARMING HER UP, PART TWO

Finger play	Inserting two or three fingers into the woman's vagina, the man uses his thumb to rub her clitoris. Alternating pressure and using deep thrusting movements or vibration adds intensity.
G-spot play	Inserting two fingers into the woman's vagina, the G-spot is only a short way in, against the front wall of the vagina. The man can rub and stroke her G-spot while stimulating her clitoris with his thumb.

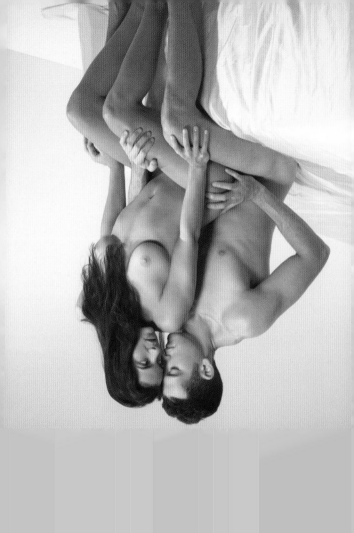

The man sits up straight—on the edge of a bed or chair—pulling the woman, who is facing away from him, on top of him by her waist. He puts his lingam into her yoni and she rides him. The Kama Sutra says that the loins and thighs should slap together, like the sound of an "elephant's ears."

SEDUCTIONS

This position is perfect for role-playing.

The man could pretend to be a rock star or king while the woman is the adoring fan or hapless maiden wandering by. He pulls her to his lap and begins to thrust into her before she even realizes what is happening. Her lust grows as she tries to watch his face. He is taken with the beauty of her flesh as he pulls her down on him. She can try to get away as he keeps pulling her back. She can sink into his lap, slowly moving her hips and kissing his face. The man can play with her breasts, tweaking her nipples or rolling them in his fingers. He can pull her hair back with one hand, telling her how delicious she feels, as his other hand grinds her down onto his hips.

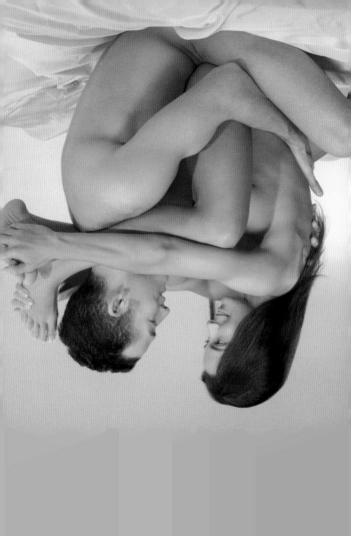

The man and woman sit face-to-face. The man sits with his legs bent and the bottoms of his feet pressed together. The woman wraps her legs around the man's neck—with the help of the man—and holds her toes with her hands while he penetrates her.

SEDUCTIONS

This position requires flexibility. People with back or leg problems or who are overweight should not attempt The Lotus. For women with large breasts, adjustments may need to be made to get comfortable.

GETTING READY

Personal hygiene is always important—whether for matters of love or career. When you look and smell good, you feel good.

Always try to take at least a quick shower before you have sexual relations. Keep your personal grooming habits under control, however, as date night shouldn't mean a two-hour preparation.

Keep hair clean and trimmed. Men should remember that a five o'clock shadow can be rough on a woman's delicate flesh. And women should keep their legs clean-shaven, as well. These days, the trend is for both men and women to shave or wax at least part of their pubic hair, if not all. Furthermore, more and more men are waxing their chests and arms.

Feel free to do whatever works best for you and your partner, even if that means doing nothing at all. It's important to discuss with your partner what turns both of you on—and off. Some women like their men hairy, while others prefer the smooth, clean feeling of a bare chest. Likewise, some men prefer hairy armpits or legs on a woman. In the end, pleasing your partner (and yourself!) is what matters most.

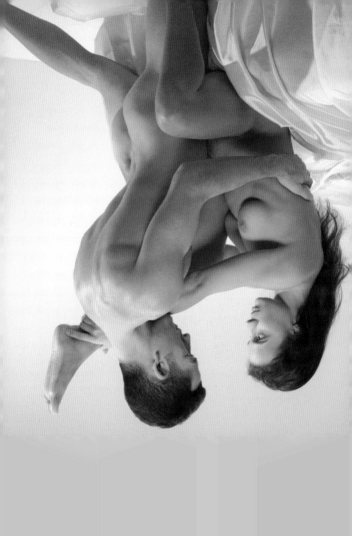

The woman sits on the edge of a bed or chair and raises one leg vertically, as straight as she can, so that it is pointing out in front of her. The man kneels or squats before her as he enters her. He will likely have to hold the balance for both himself and the woman, as she will have only one leg on the floor for support.

SEDUCTIONS

The Peacock position illustrated has been modified to represent a more realistic pose that more women will be capable of performing (i.e., her raised leg is bent and rests on the man's shoulder).

The woman needs to remember to breathe deeply and keep her muscles relaxed as she holds her leg up. To protect his knees, the man can put pillows on the floor and for balance, he can wrap his arm around her leg as he penetrates her. To make this position more erotic, the partners should stare into each other's eyes.

TRAINING EXERCISE

Stretching is always a good idea, even if you're not planning to do anything particularly adventurous in the bedroom. Try doing lunges and splits while you're sitting around or watching television. Do lunges facing forward and to the side. While doing a split—whether to the front or the side—remember to breathe into the stretch.

In addition, practice kicks, which will not only tone you, but will increase your flexibility. As a challenge, set weekly goals for how high you can kick and how many kicks you can do.

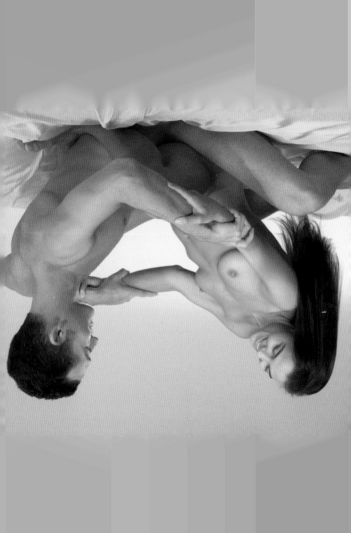

The man and women start sitting face-to-face, breast to chest. The lovers wrap their legs around each other and lock their own heels together. The man puts his lingam into the woman's yoni and they clasp each other's wrists and lean back.

In this position, the man and woman can pull each other back and forth, like a game of seesaw. The movement should be gentle and smooth. Stare into each other's eyes and enjoy the rocking sensation.

SEDUCTIONS

Communication is the key to a lasting and loving relationship, as is trust. Many of the positions of the Kama Sutra can leave one of the partners feeling vulnerable, so it is always important that both partners feel safe and secure with one another. If there are hidden resentments or hang-ups, the experience won't be as joyful or fulfilling.

Learning how to talk to each other about sex is vitally important. Learning how to listen and acknowledging your partner are equally important.

Try to keep the bedroom a safe place, where talking about sexuality or fantasies won't lead to larger issues and insecurities. If one partner is uncomfortable with something the other person wants to try, talk it out. Find out why he or she is uncomfortable. It could simply be an irrational fear, or perhaps there was a bad experience associated with the act. Either way, open communication is essential to satisfy any sexual relationship.

For example, some people dislike oral sex. Sometimes it's because they think it's dirty or degrading. Others may have had bad experiences. Sometimes just talking about it and being open with each other can turn the situation around.

If a person isn't willing to try something new (for whatever reason), let it go. Find something else you can agree on and move forward.

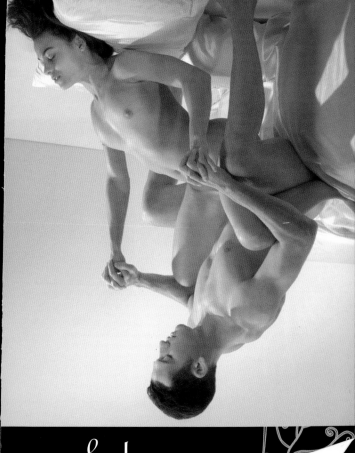

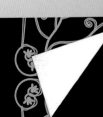

The Trapeze

The man sits on the edge of the bed as the woman faces and straddles him. He puts his lingam into her yoni as they hold hands. Slowly, the woman leans back until she is hanging upside down. For balance, she can hook her legs around the man's thighs.

SEDUCTIONS

Until this position is mastered, it will no doubt bring a lot of laughter.

Putting pillows on the floor can help nervous women be more relaxed as they lean back. The man must hold the woman firmly and confidently so she trusts he won't drop her. The woman should be careful not to slide along the floor, which could cause them to lose balance. If there are loose throw rugs or slippery wooden floors, try this position somewhere with more traction.

The Trapeze won't work well if the man is thin and the woman is heavy. For success with this position, the man must be strong enough to hold the woman's full body weight in case she slips.

GETTING READY

Bedroom talk should be open and honest and filled with compliments. Some people believe discussing sexual issues should be done outside of the bedroom. However, when issues are approached with tact and in the right manner, they can be addressed almost anywhere.

Try wording any issue you have in a positive tone while encouraging your partner to try something else instead (rather than continuing with whatever is bothering you). For example, rather than saying, "Don't touch me like that," try saying, "I wonder what it would be like if you gently licked my clitoris while putting your fingers inside of my vagina."

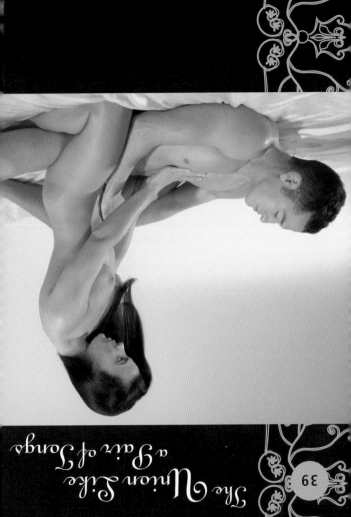

The Union Like a Pair of Tongs

The man lies on his back, keeping his legs straight or slightly bent. The woman sits on top of him, with one leg on either side of him, while she puts his lingam into her yoni, squeezing and milking him.

SEDUCTIONS

This is a great position to use when the man is tired from other positions. The woman can use as much energy as she desires, rocking gently on him, or riding him up and down. The purpose of this position is for the woman to squeeze and release his lingam. For added tightness, she can squeeze her thighs as well.

An elephant partnered with a hare (see #9) may find that milking the lingam isn't too successful. With a few alterations, however, this position may work better than most for a couple of this nature. Try putting a pillow beneath the man's hips. If it's more comfortable, the man can keep a pillow under his head as well and he can play with her breasts.

This is a great position for the woman to show her dominance, as well as for her to be affectionate and nurturing towards her man. The woman can rub his shoulders and biceps, stroke his chest, and play with or lick and bite his nipples. She can also try different scratching techniques on the man's torso and arms.

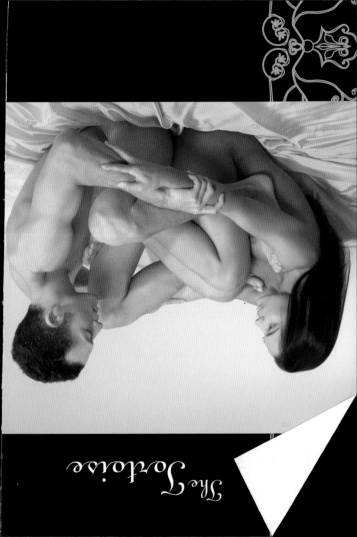

The Tortoise

The man and woman sit face-to-face. The man plays with the woman's breasts using his feet while the woman pushes her feet against the man's chest. The man pushes forward with his thighs to place his lingam in her yoni. They hold hands and gaze into one another's eyes.

SEDUCTIONS

This position is advanced and requires a great deal of flexibility. In positions such as The Tortoise, the yoga influence of the culture is very apparent.

Another way to try this position is for the man to sit in a lotus, or cross-legged, position. The woman then sits in his lap and they press their chests together. The lovers have their heads together—eye to eye, lips to lips.

The idea of The Tortoise is for the man and woman to mirror each other, providing energy flow between the partners. Try to concentrate on where the energy in your body is flowing and imagine it flowing into your lover. Visualize a constant flow of energy uniting you both.

GETTING READY

Although a nice steak dinner and a bottle of wine may seem like a great idea, try to eat lightly if lovemaking is on the agenda for the evening.

Foods that inspire love include fruits, chocolate, sweets, and oysters. Bring some melted chocolate and whipped cream to bed and decorate each other. Feeding one another is erotic, and the receiver always feels like royalty.

[Note: Remember to never insert food into a yoni as it can cause infections and/or other problems.]

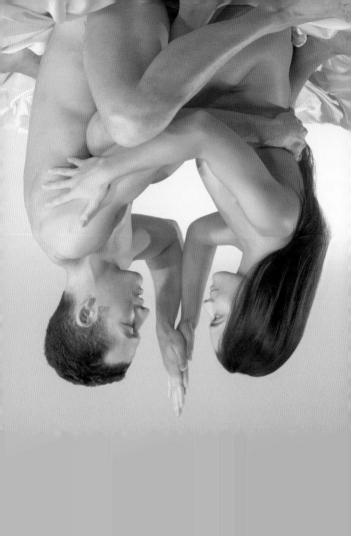

The man and woman sit face-to-face. The woman raises one hand in the air and wraps her corresponding leg around the man's waist. Mirroring her, the man places his hand against her hand in the air. He wraps his leg around her waist in the same manner, putting his lingam into her yoni. If possible, they each lift the foot of their other leg into the air, placing them on each other (not illustrated). They "peddle" against each other's feet while staring into each other's eyes.

SEDUCTIONS

This position is great fun to try, but only the most flexible partners will be able to both put their feet up against the other for peddling—and perform intercourse at the same time.

GETTING READY

Women take longer then men to become aroused. The man can help by being gentle, charming, and complimentary. Little things, like opening the door or bringing her flowers can go a long way. He should touch his woman while listening to her and be generous with the compliments.

In lovemaking, a pleasant, relaxing, sensual atmosphere goes a long way. It's always nice to keep fresh flowers out and to burn some incense. Playing romantic music in the background can also enhance the mood, and offering a foot or shoulder massage can help to connect physically.

Most importantly, a woman must feel she can trust her man. She needs to trust that he really is a kind, gentle man and she needs to trust that his desire is only for her.

Some couples have problems sending signals to each other, so small acts of affection can go a long way in showing love.

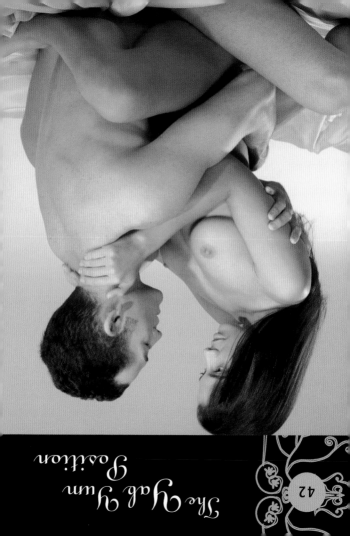

The Yab Yum Position

42

The man sits either with his legs loosely crossed or straight out in front of him with the woman sitting in his lap. He places his lingam into her yoni and she wraps her legs around his waist. They can wrap their arms around each other, or they can lean back slightly to stare into each other's eyes.

WARMING HIM UP

Despite what many women may think, men need foreplay as well. Some men are turned on by just the sight of a naked woman and are ready to go. Some men need to turn off their brains and wind down from work or other concerns before they can begin to think about sex. Speaking soothingly to your man and giving lots of compliments will help ease him down.

Women should learn how to respect and enjoy a man's lingam—it's not just a matter of grabbing and pulling on it a few times to get him in the mood. Remember eye contact is always important. Throw in some pleasingly dirty talk, and above all, show enthusiasm.

As an aside, some men enjoy having their testicles and scrotum tugged, pulled, cupped, and caressed, while other men dislike having their testicles touched at all. Some men prefer that only their penis or testicles be touched at a certain time, and some men love having everything touched at the same time. Be certain to ask what turns your man on so that you can provide him with maximum stimulation.

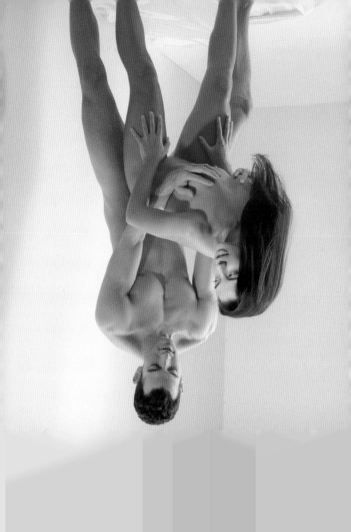

The woman stands with legs apart and her hands on her thighs. The man stands behind her, placing his lingam into her yoni, holding her at the waist, shoulders, or breasts.

SEDUCTIONS

This is a good "quickie" position that can be performed easily and in many situations.

The woman can squeeze and contract her yoni to provide more stimulation for the man's lingam. She can arch her back to change sensations as she looks back at her man, turning him on more.

The man can squeeze the woman's breasts, or enjoy them as they flop and hit his hands as he holds her sides. He can enjoy watching as his lingam enters the yoni. To give him a greater sense of power, he can pull her hair backand wrap it around his hand.

GETTING HIM READY

To take your man's mind off his worries, and to steer him towards a night of passion, treat him like a king. Wear an outfit he enjoys seeing you in, or tease him by wearing only a bra and panties. Men enjoy "peek-a-boo" attire, which piques their curiosity, imagination, and urge to hunt.

Remove his shoes and massage his feet with scented lotions. Remember, there are many erogenous spots on the foot, so be certain to hit every inch. Massage his shoulders and knead his back muscles. Feed him oysters, strawberries dipped in chocolate, or other tasty treats while wiping his mouth daintily with a napkin. All of these serve to help the man relax and feel important, appreciated, and desired.

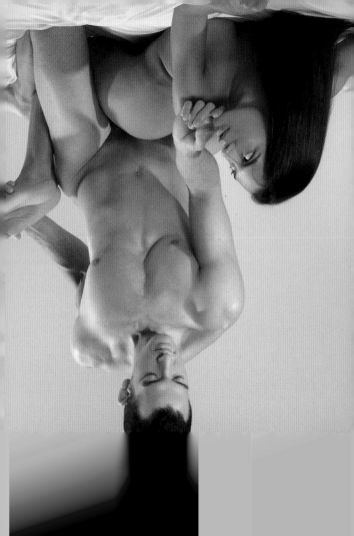

The woman lies on her stomach while the man holds both her ankles in one hand. He touches her chin with the other hand. He kneels or squats, with his legs straddling her, as he penetrates her.

SEDUCTIONS

This position sounds complicated, and though it isn't easy, it isn't impossible either.

The woman should roll around on the bed, playfully purring, and writhing like a big cat, as she lifts her hips to receive him, arching her back to provide friction.

The man will enjoy watching her body undulate as she plays. He can capture his woman by stroking her face and hair, coaxing her to let him enter her.

FOOT PLAY

Feet are an oft-overlooked erogenous zone. While some people love feet or even have a foot fetish, other people may find feet to be gross. But feet can provide some magnificent pleasures. However, it's always important to remember that a clean foot is a must—and to always keep toenails trimmed. A bath, shower, or even a foot soak not only feels great, but will soften the skin and prepare the foot for a lovely massage.

Rub oils or lotion on each other's feet. Take the foot in your lap, and knead it firmly, paying attention to the pads of the feet, heels, and ankles, and pulling gently on each toe. The spots between the toes are great acupuncture triggers, so take care to rub them gently.

For added sensation and sensuality, suck on each other's toes.

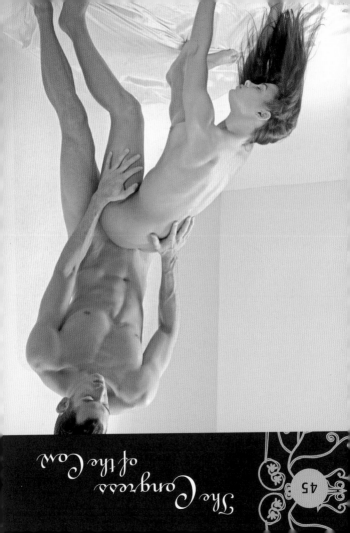

The Congress of the Cow

The woman stands with her legs apart, bending at the waist to place her hands on floor. The man stands behind her, placing his lingam into her yoni. He can put his hands on her breasts, hips, or thighs.

SEDUCTIONS

This is a great position for the shower, the office, or any other odd place a couple may find themselves. You can even try this position in the woods, where the woman can use a fallen log or stump for support.

REVVING HIS ENGINE

Sparking the Fire   Using a water-based lubricant or lotion, the woman rubs the lingam gently between both hands, as if she is trying to start a fire.

———

Warming the Head   Holding the lingam at the base of the shaft, the woman strokes, rubs, and cups the head with her other hand.

———

Belly Pat   With the man lying down, the woman cups his testicles with one hand, while using the other hand to stroke and pet the underside of the man's lingam as it lies against his belly.

———

Stroking the Shaft   The woman grasps the lingam at the top, slides her hand down the shaft, and releases her hand at the bottom. She repeats this with her other hand and then continues at the bottom. She repeats this with her other hand and then continues the entire motion motion several times, trying different speeds and pressures.

[Note: Using lots of lubricant will be more pleasurable for him. Trying to stroke a lingam without lubricant can be painful for some men. Find out which strokes your man enjoys the most. You can do this by asking him what strokes he uses on himself.

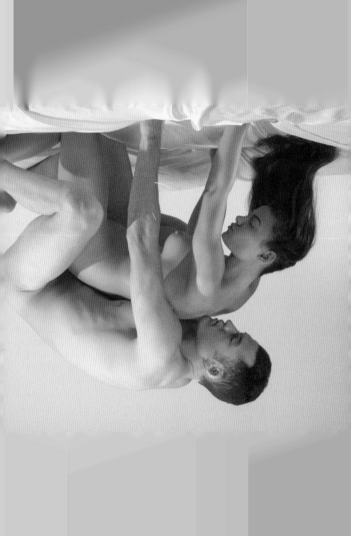

The woman goes on her hands and knees and the man can either squat or kneel behind her as he places his lingam into her yoni. The woman creates movement by arching her back.

SEDUCTIONS

This position is one of the many animal-like positions in the Kama Sutra where lovers should let go of inhibitions and embrace their primitive instincts. Deer rut vigorously and noisily, and this position is supposed to inspire such play.

The Rutting of the Deer is more forceful, vigorous, and rough than other rear-entry positions. This position is often used as a final—or finishing-up—position for many couples. The Rutting of the Deer is often mistakenly referred to as "doggie style," when, in fact, many couples naturally make transitions between doggie- and deer-positions as part of their regular sexual routine (see #47 for more on The Dog position).

In this position, the man is to thrust into the woman as fast and forcefully as he can as the woman meets his thrusts by arching her back. The man can hold her by her hips, waist, or breasts, or he may also support himself with his hands on the bed, nipping or biting his woman's back and shoulders.

In many of the rear-entry positions, the G-spot is nicely stimulated, but the clitoris is often neglected. To add more punch to the position, the man can use his fingers to stimulate her clitoris—or she can stimulate herself. A bullet-style vibrator or the strap-on "butterfly" type vibrator can help to stimulate the clitoris while the G-spot is being manipulated.

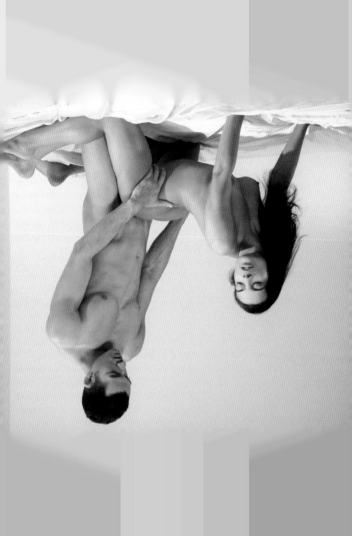

The woman kneels with her hands and knees on the bed and her legs spread slightly. The man kneels behind her, his knees between hers, gripping her waist as he penetrates her. The woman twists around to meet his eyes.

SEDUCTIONS

The best way for a couple to know the difference between The Dog and The Rutting of the Deer (see #46) is that The Dog is a slower, more intimate movement. There is eye contact in The Dog position as the woman turns to gaze at her man.

The man can hold the woman's hips, buttocks, thighs, breasts, or shoulders as he thrusts into her. The Dog position allows the man to enjoy looking at his woman as his lingam penetrates her yoni.

To create different angles for penetration, the woman can arch her back up or down or use pillows under her pelvis and hips to help prop her up—this is especially important and useful if she has knee or wrist problems. Planting pillows or cushions under her pelvis can also be a good source of friction to stimulate her clitoris.

If the man takes his time penetrating her, he can find and stimulate her G-spot until she ejaculates. Always be certain to have extra towels on hand if this happens.

As the man grows more vigorous, he can wrap her hair around his hand, gently tugging on it to create a different sensation, as well as a sense of masculine power.

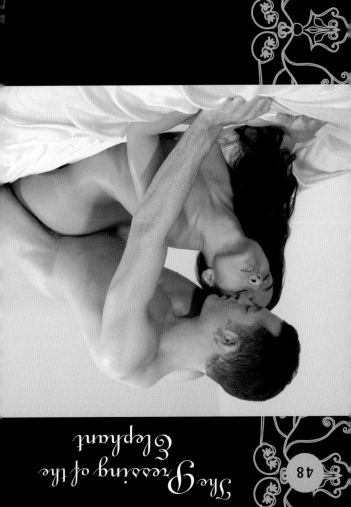

The Pleasing of the
Elephant

48

The woman lies on her stomach with her legs slightly apart, her pelvis lifted slightly so that the man can enter her. The man lies flat over her, supporting himself on his arms, with his legs on the outside of her legs as he enters her.

SEDUCTIONS

The Pressing of the Elephant allows for full-body closeness. The position is named for the animal, and isn't intended to refer to the woman's yoni or anyone's body size.

This is a slow and sensual position that is great in the morning, or when both partners are tired. The lazy, yet erotic pulse of this position brings a sense of closeness.

The man can brace himself up on his arms to kiss and nibble on his woman's cheeks, eyes, ears, and neck. Slow sensuous nips, licks, and sucks can be highly arousing for both partners. He can also clasp his hands over hers, giving him a greater sense of dominance.

The woman can push herself up on her bended arms, tossing her head back, much like an elephant. As she pushes her head up, she can expose her neck and shoulder area for her man to kiss, suck, nibble, and nuzzle her. She can put pillows under her pelvis to raise her hips higher to meet her man and she can tilt her back or stick up her buttocks for deeper penetration.

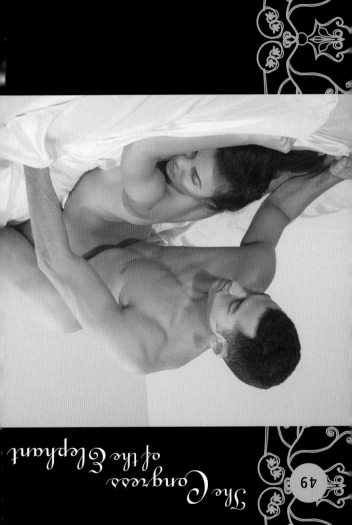

The Congress of the Elephant

49

The woman lies on her stomach with her legs out, pressing her head, breasts, and arms into the bed. She raises her buttocks into the air so the man can enter her. The man lies atop her, his chest to her back as he enters her from behind.

SEDUCTIONS

The woman can place pillows under her pelvis so her yoni is better angled to receive the man's lingam, or she can push her forehead into the bed while thrusting her buttocks into the air. When the lingam is in the woman's yoni, she can squeeze her thighs tightly together. This provides more sensation for the man, especially around his scrotum. She can reach down and stimulate her clitoris with her fingers and tighten and release her pelvic muscles while the man's lingam is inside of her. Lovers can also wrap their feet around each other, clasp hands or intertwine fingers.

If the man is heavy, he should keep his weight on his hands and legs, and be aware if his stomach is pushing into the woman. He should be cautious of how much body weight he is putting on the woman. This position is great for closeness and for pressing together as tightly as possible, but be careful to avoid squeezing too hard or hurting. The man's chest should not touch the woman's back, so that she can breathe easily.

For a highly erotic game, the woman can pretend to be asleep while the man takes her.

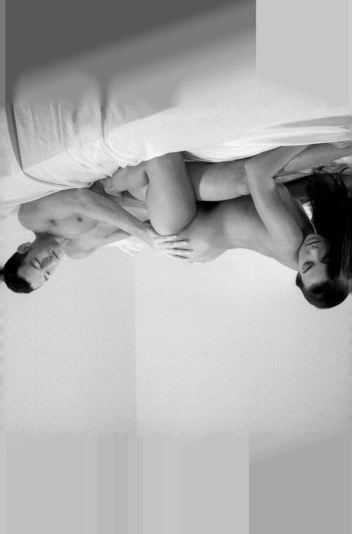

The man lies on his back with the woman crouching over him and facing away. She holds herself on her hands and knees while placing his lingam in her yoni. Her hands rest on either side of his legs and her legs wrap against his sides for support.

SEDUCTIONS

Inversion provides the man with a delicious view of his woman's buttocks, as well as the excitement of watching his lingam thrusting in and out of her yoni. He can enjoy her buttocks in many ways: squeezing, pulling, kneading, pinching, slapping, or spanking them. With her consent, he can even use a paddle or whip across her buttocks, or he can play with her anus by inserting a finger or sex toy into it.

Using pillows under his shoulders and neck, the man can also lie helplessly and let the woman do all the work. The woman can squeeze and tighten her yoni, milking his lingam. She can squeeze her yoni and hold her thighs together so that he is unable to pull out—making him harder if he's starting to go soft. If the woman feels that he is going to come too soon, she can stop the movement and wait for him to cool down by rocking back and forth gently on her hands and knees, or by swinging or gyrating her hips in a circle. For balance, she can hold his feet.

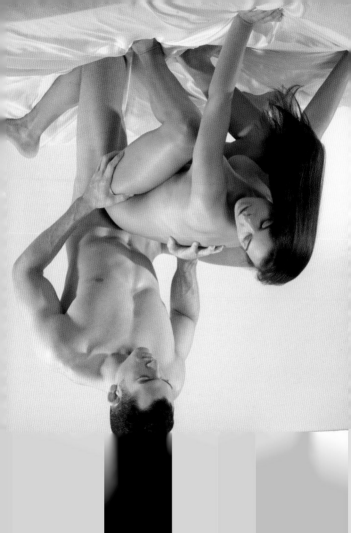

The man kneels on the bed as the woman squats back into his lap. The man bends her forward until her breasts are pushed against her thighs and he enters her.

SEDUCTIONS

This position may take some balancing to master. For support, the woman may want to use her hands on the bed or the man can hold onto the woman's hips, buttocks, thighs, or back to help move her.

The woman can try leaning back into the man and squeezing her yoni. By opening or closing her legs, lovers can see which friction works best.

As with any of the positions of the Kama Sutra, it is best to experiment with what works for the both of you and your body types. Larger women may not be able to do this position and men with larger stomachs may not have room for a woman on their laps.

TRAINING EXERCISE

Both men and woman should be limber and flexible when attempting to try some of the more adventurous Kama Sutra moves. This includes having a good sense of balance.

Imagine there is a string coming out of the top of your head, pulling you up—feel your spine elongate and your lungs fill with air. Tighten your abdominal muscles and buttocks for added balance.

To practice balancing techniques, stand up straight and lift one leg out in front of you, as high as possible.

While standing straight, lift a leg behind you and bend over as far as you can go, putting your arms out to help with weight distribution.

These simple exercises will help you learn where your center is and you'll quickly find that keeping your balance body-wise will help you in all aspects of life.

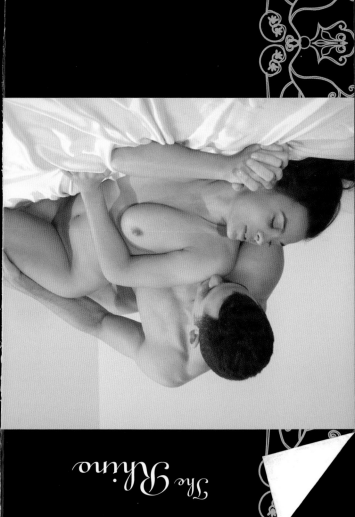

The woman lies on her side, facing away from the man as he enters her from behind.

SEDUCTIONS

This position is likely familiar to most couples who have been together for a while. The Rhino is a great lazy morning, slow, and sensual position. Some people may consider this seemingly simple position boring, but it can be quite erotic and satisfying, especially when foreplay is involved.

Using long, firm strokes along the woman's body, the man should kiss her shoulders, back, cheek, breasts, hips, and waist—moving from her thighs to her face.

He may wish to press against the back of her, while his hand reaches around to her front to manipulate her clitoris. This position works best if the man continues to manipulate the woman's clitoris while he is inside of her. Breathing lightly into the woman's ear or whispering naughty ideas can also be highly erotic.

© 2015 Quarto Publishing Group USA Inc.

Text and photography © 2007 by Quiver

First published in 2015 by Quiver,
an imprint of The Quarto Group.
100 Cummings Center, Suite 265-D,
Beverly, MA 01915, USA.
T (978) 282-9590 F (978) 283-2742
www.QuartoKnows.com

Quiver titles are also available at discount for retail, wholesale, promotional, and
bulk purchase. For details, contact the Special Sales Manager by email at special-
sales@quarto.com or by mail at The Quarto Group, Attn: Special Sales Manager,
401 Second Avenue North, Suite 310, Minneapolis, MN 55401 USA.

The Publisher maintains the records relating to images in this book required by
18 USC 2257. Records are located at The Quarto Group, 100 Cummings Center,
Suite 265-D, Beverly, MA 01915, USA.

19   12 13 14 15

ISBN: 978-1-59233-664-7

Library of Congress Cataloging-in-Publication Data available

Cover design by traffic

Photography by Chermus Photography

Printed and bound in Hong Kong

Brimming with creative inspiration, how-to projects, and useful
information to enrich your everyday life, Quarto Knows is a favorite
destination for those pursuing their interests and passions. Visit our
site and dig deeper with our books into your area of interest:
Quarto Creates, Quarto Cooks, Quarto Homes, Quarto Lives,
Quarto Drives, Quarto Explores, Quarto Gifts, or Quarto Kids.